@RosenTeenTalk

ADDICTIONS

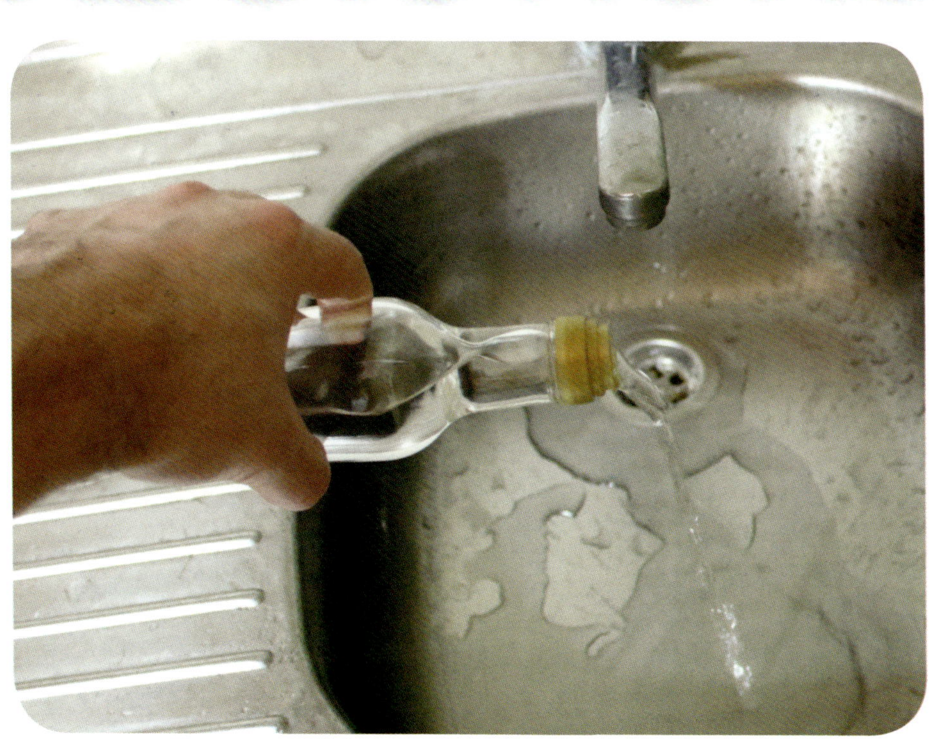

Ryan Wolf

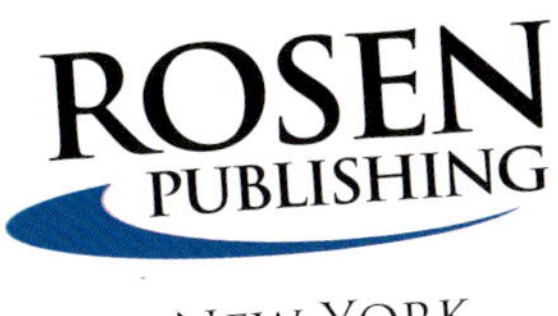

NEW YORK

Published in 2021 by The Rosen Publishing Group, Inc.
29 East 21st Street, New York, NY 10010

First Edition

Editor: Theresa Emminizer
Designer: Michael Flynn
Interior Layout: Rachel Rising

Photo Credits: Cover, p. 1 Far700/Shutterstock.com; Cover, pp. 1, 3,5, 45 Motortion Films/Shutterstock.com; Cover, Cosmic_Design/Shutterstock.com; Cover, pp. 1,6,8,12,14,18,20,22,24,26,28,32,34,36,38,40,42 Vitya_M/ Shutterstock.com; pp. 3,11 Piotr Wawrzyniuk/Shutterstock.com; pp. 3,17 Juanmonino/ E+/Getty Images; pp. 3,31 Anton27/Shutterstock.com; pp. 3, 40 Hugo Felix/Shutterstock.com;com; p. 6 azurek/Shutterstock.com; p. 8 GrAl/Shutterstock.com; p. 9 Daniel Heighton/Shutterstock.com; p.12 Igor Normann/Shutterstock.com; p. 13 TAW4/Shutterstock.com; pp. 15, 29 Photographee.eu/Shutterstock.com; p. 18 Sharon Mccutcheon/ EyeEm/Getty Images; p. 19 Oleksandrum/Shutterstock.com; p. 20 krisanapong detraphiphat/ Moment/Getty Images; p. 21 5 second Studio/Shutterstock.com; p. 22 sruilk/Shutterstock.com; p. 23 Lifestyle discover/Shutterstock.com; p. 25 Victor Moussa/Shutterstock.com; p. 26 archielv/Shutterstock.com; p. 27 Ken Weinrich/Shutterstock.com; p. 32 namtipStudio/Shutterstock.com; p. 33 Digital Storm/Shutterstock.com; p. 34 JJFarq/Shutterstock.com; p. 35 Neveshkin Nikolay/Shutterstock.com; p. 36 Peter Byrne - PA Images / Contributor/Getty Images; p. 37 CLS Digital Arts/ Shutterstock.com; p. 38 KARRASTOCK/ Moment/Getty Images; p. 39 SDI Productions/ E+/Getty Images; p. 41 Eivaisla/ Shutterstock.com; p.43 Maksim Shmeljov/Shutterstock.

Library of Congress Cataloging-in-Publication Data

Names: Wolf, Ryan, author.
Title: Addictions / Ryan Wolf.
Description: New York : Rosen Publishing, [2021] | Series: @RosenTeenTalk | Includes index.
Identifiers: LCCN 2020000900 | ISBN 9781499467949 (paperback) | ISBN 9781499467956 (library binding)
Subjects: LCSH: Compulsive behavior--Juvenile literature. | Substance abuse--Juvenile literature.
Classification: LCC RC533 .W65 2021 | DDC 616.86--dc23
LC record available at https://lccn.loc.gov/2020000900

Manufactured in the United States of America

CPSIA Compliance Information: Batch #BSR20. For further information contact Rosen Publishing, New York, New York at 1-800-237-9932.

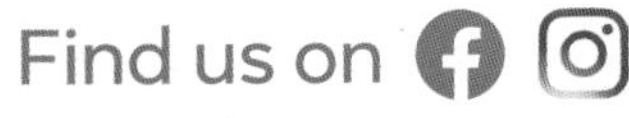

CONTENTS

Chapter 1

How Much Is Too Much?

My friend Max used to hang out with me every week. We'd play video games and watch sports together. This past summer, he started partying with some older kids. They like to get drunk and smoke weed. Sometimes they even pop pills they steal from their parents. Max talks about how fun it is to feel so free. But now it seems like he can't stop getting high.

A few months ago, we started tenth grade. Max likes to skip class and he never gets his homework done. Whenever I see him, he looks tired. He always smells like smoke and his eyes are bloodshot. I don't judge Max for his choices. But I'm worried about him. Will he always be like this?

In the United States, about 21 million people struggle with addiction to alcohol and illegal drugs.

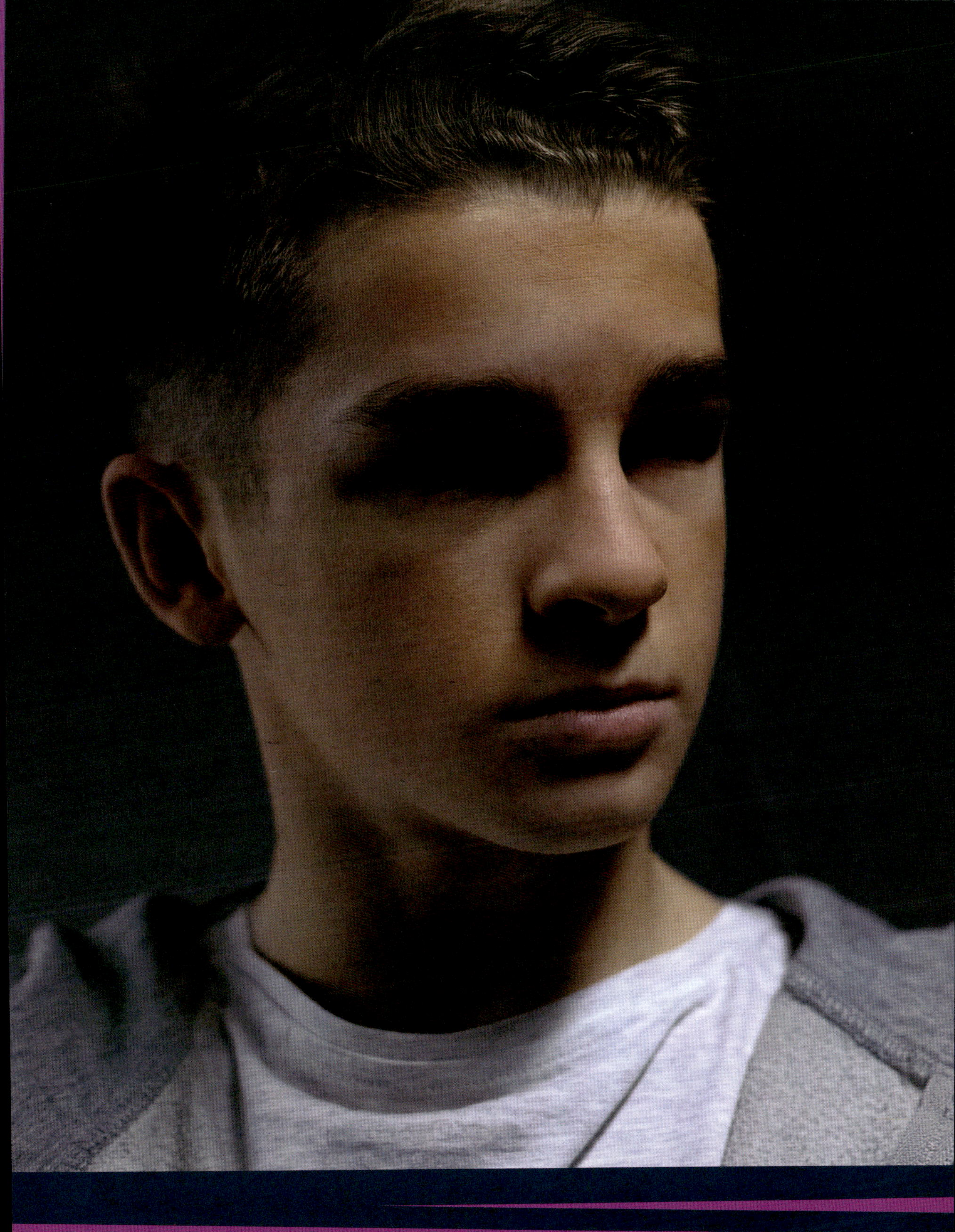

WHAT IS ADDICTION?

Addiction is a disease, or illness. It's caused by habits that affect the brain's reward system. Addiction makes people lose their impulse control. This means it's very hard for addicts to stop their behaviors and habits. They often do things without thinking. Some addicts will feel sick or deeply unhappy if they do not obey their cravings, or wants.

Addiction can make people feel trapped, ashamed, and alone. Always remember that there are people out there who understand and can offer a path forward.

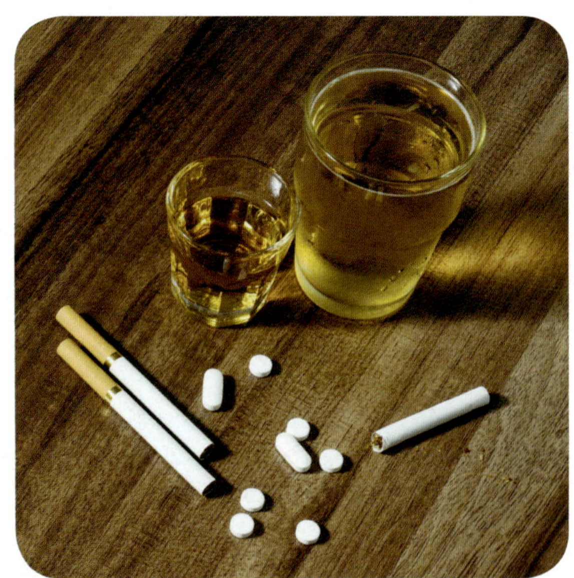

People can be addicted to almost anything. But some drugs and activities are more addictive than others. It's important to reach out to caring professionals if you feel like a habit or behavior is out of control.

THERE IS HOPE!

While it might seem impossible, many people overcome their addictions with help and support. There are resources, or helpful aids, for people who struggle with many different kinds of addiction.

Things that can greatly help with addiction include:

- **Crisis** counseling
- **Detoxing**
- Friendly check-ins
- One-on-one therapy, or treatment
- Professional treatment and **rehabilitation** (rehab)
- Relaxation practices
- **Sober** living communities
- Special medicines given by a doctor
- Support groups

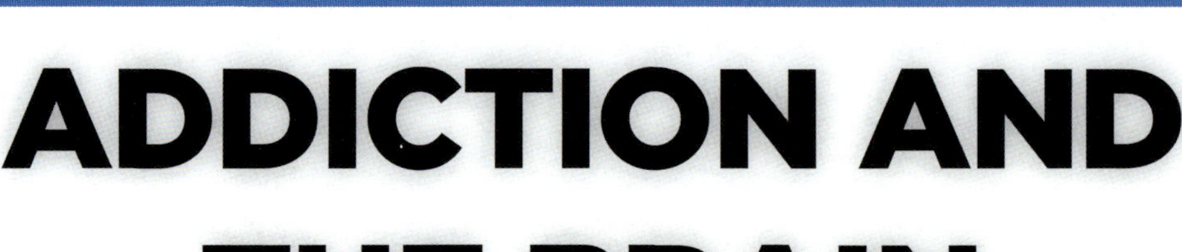

ADDICTION AND THE BRAIN

Addiction starts because of changes to the brain. A chemical called **dopamine** gives the body pleasure. Dopamine is also tied to memory and learning. This makes it easy for the body to remember which activities gave it pleasure.

Dopamine is a chemical that has many different roles, or uses. When it travels to the brain's "pleasure center," it makes the body feel good.

How does an addiction start?

1) Dopamine is sent out during activities like eating, drinking, sex, and drug use.

2) The most addictive drugs and activities create powerful blasts of dopamine. The chemicals travel on a path called the **reward circuit**.

3) When an addictive activity is done enough times, the brain starts needing more and more.

4) If addicts try to stop doing what their brains want, they might get dangerously sick or emotionally upset.

Over time, the brain lets out less dopamine in response to a **trigger**. This makes addicted people want even more of the drugs or activities they enjoy. At some point, they will seek out things they are addicted to even if they no longer get any pleasure from them.

Chapter 2

ALCOHOL ABUSE

I used to get a buzz after a couple of drinks. Now it takes four or five to get me there. After I start feeling good, I can't stop drinking. I want to keep the buzz going or take it to the next level. So I drink more and more until I puke or pass out.

In the morning, I feel like dying. I'm so weak. I can barely even reach the toilet to throw up. My head is pounding and my arms feel like heavy weights. Why do I do this to myself?

Tonight, my friends invited me over for another party. I'll probably drink myself sick all over again. What is wrong with me? Where is my self-control?

People who start drinking before age 15 have a higher chance of getting addicted to alcohol.

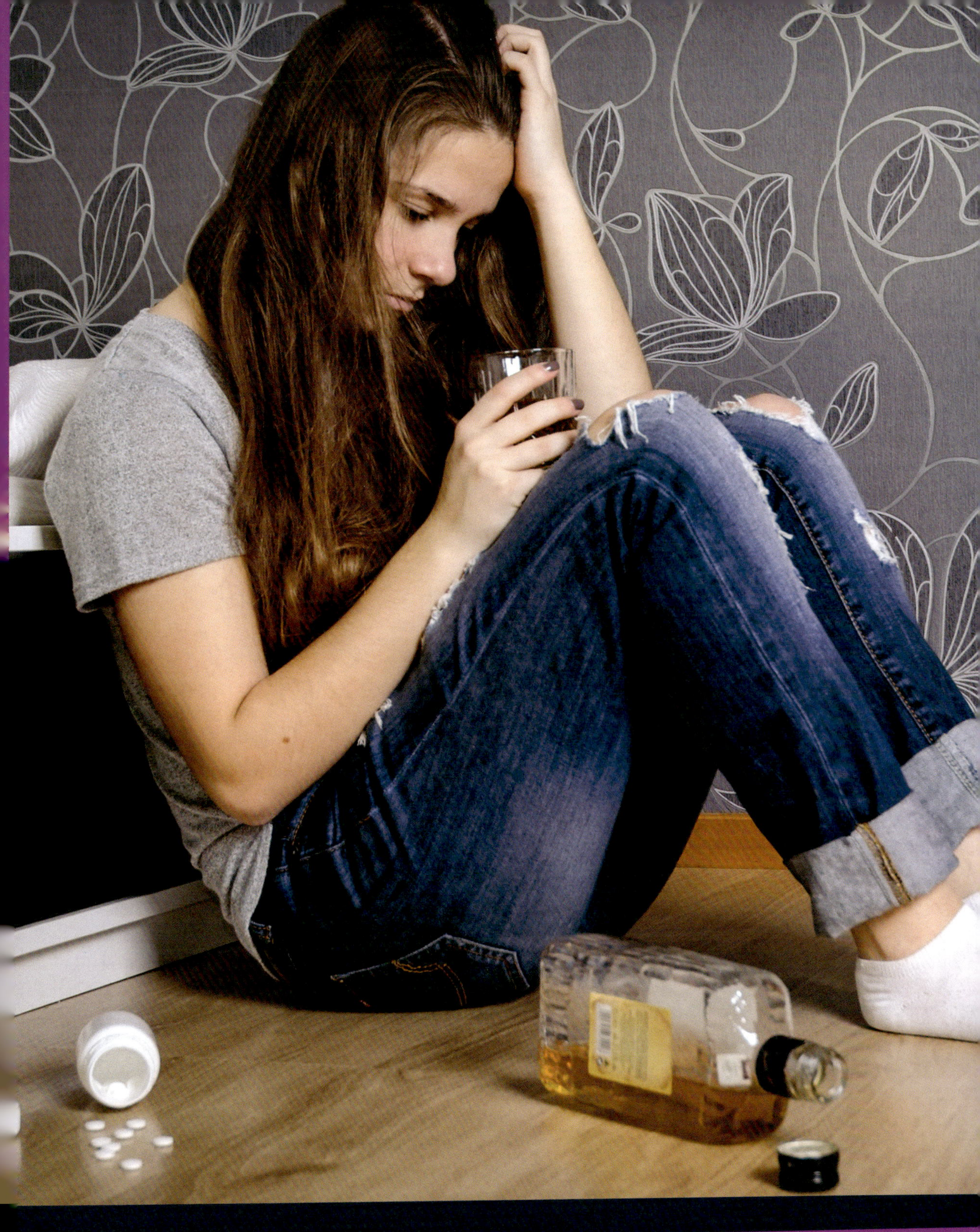

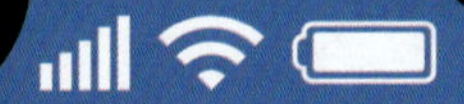

RISKS AND DANGERS

People often make bad decisions when they're drunk. Sometimes they do things that hurt others. When people decide to drive after drinking alcohol, they are more dangerous than they might think. Every day, 30 people in the United States are killed in drunk driving accidents.

More than 1 out of every 20 deaths across the world are connected to alcohol abuse.

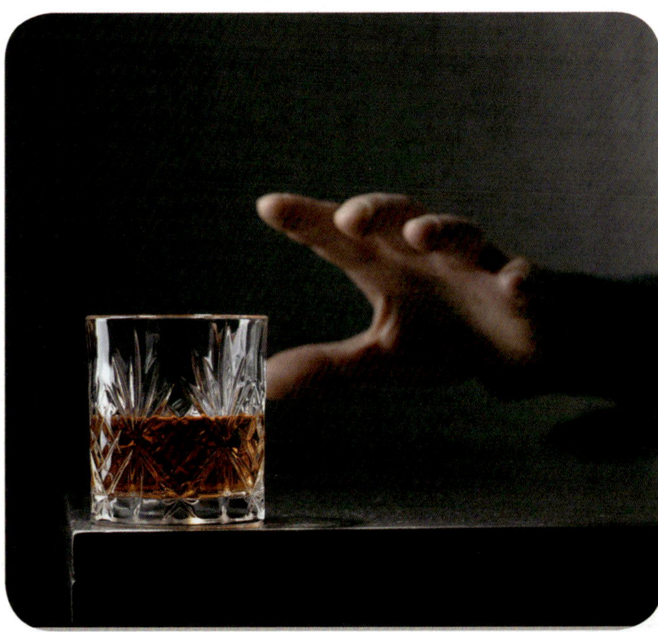

Long-term heavy drinking can create deadly liver problems and other health issues like cancer. It may also lead to an addiction to alcohol, known as alcoholism. It can harm relationships and break apart families.

DON'T DRINK AND DRIVE

Knowing when to stop drinking might save your life. Having more than four drinks in two hours can lead to alcohol poisoning.

One drink is equal to a:

- 12 oz. can of beer
- 5 oz. glass of wine
- 1.5 oz. shot of **liquor**

In many cases, alcohol poisoning makes a person throw up. If someone is sleeping or passed out, the person could choke to death while throwing up. Call 911 if you see someone who is unconscious, or passed out, from alcohol, throwing up, or breathing less than eight times per minute.

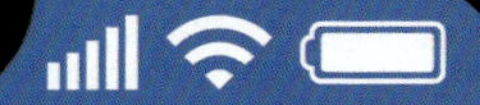

FINDING SUPPORT

If you, a friend, or a family member have trouble with alcohol abuse, you're not alone. At any time, day or night, you can reach out to these free resources:

Above the Influence

https://abovetheinfluence.com/resources

Text ABOVE to 741-741 to talk with a crisis counselor.

Boys Town National Hotline

https://www.yourlifeyourvoice.org

Text VOICE to 20121 or call 1-800-448-3000 to contact a counselor.

Substance Abuse and Mental Health Services Administration (SAMHSA)

https://www.samhsa.gov/find-help/national-helpline

Call 1-800-662-HELP (4357) to get free information about where you can go for help.

Counseling and rehabilitation can help people who struggle with alcohol. They can kick their addiction and become their best selves.

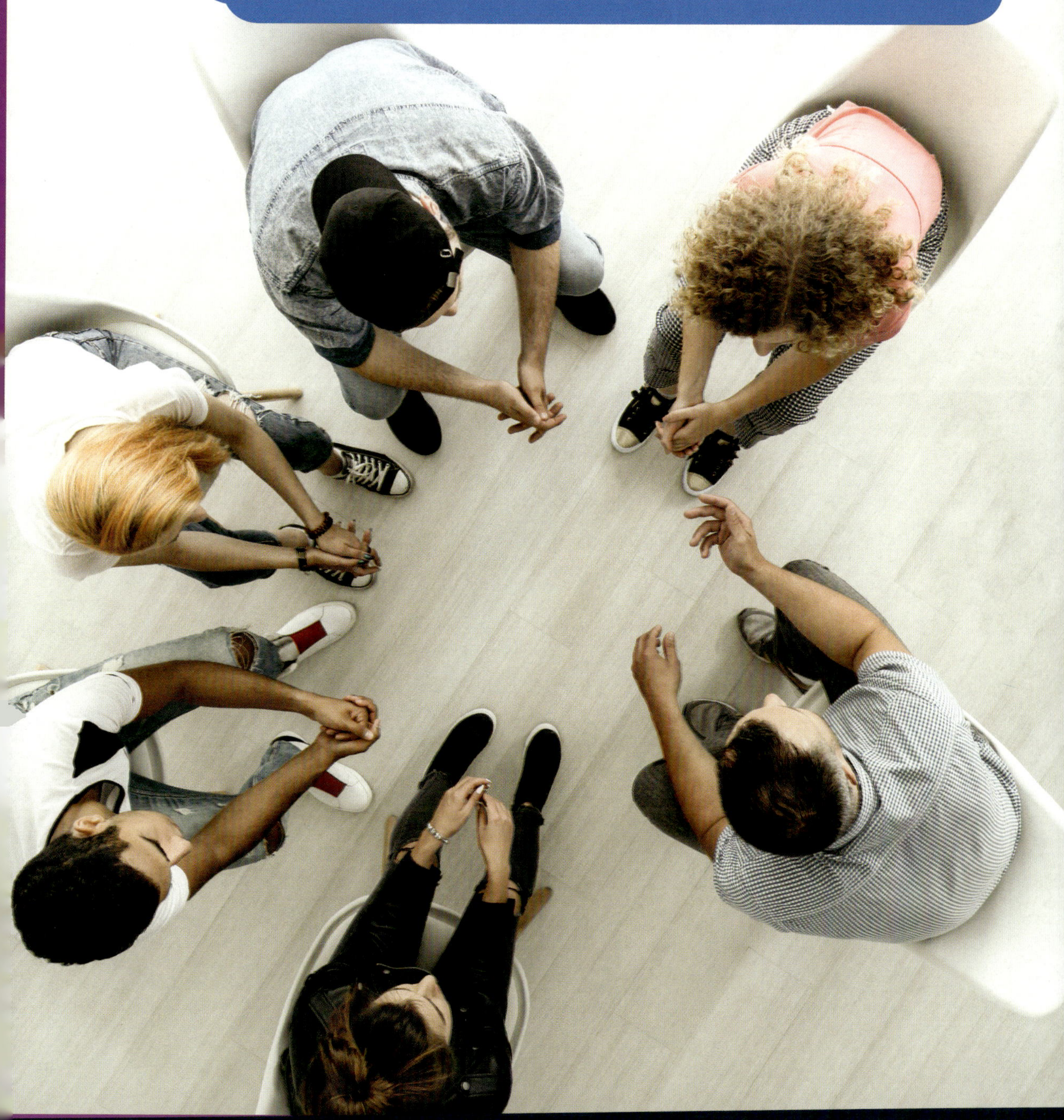

Chapter 3

DRUG ABUSE

When I started smoking pot with my friends, it made the world seem more interesting. It was freaky at first, but I got used to the feeling. Now I have my own stash and smoke all the time.

I sneak my vape into the restroom so I can get high even when I'm at school. Sometimes it's hard to pay attention in class if I get too stoned. But when I'm not high, life just seems boring.

If I get caught smoking weed at school, I'll get in huge trouble. I keep taking that risk anyway. Why is the drug so important to me? Why does it feel like I need it to be happy?

Most people who are addicted to drugs began using them while in high school.

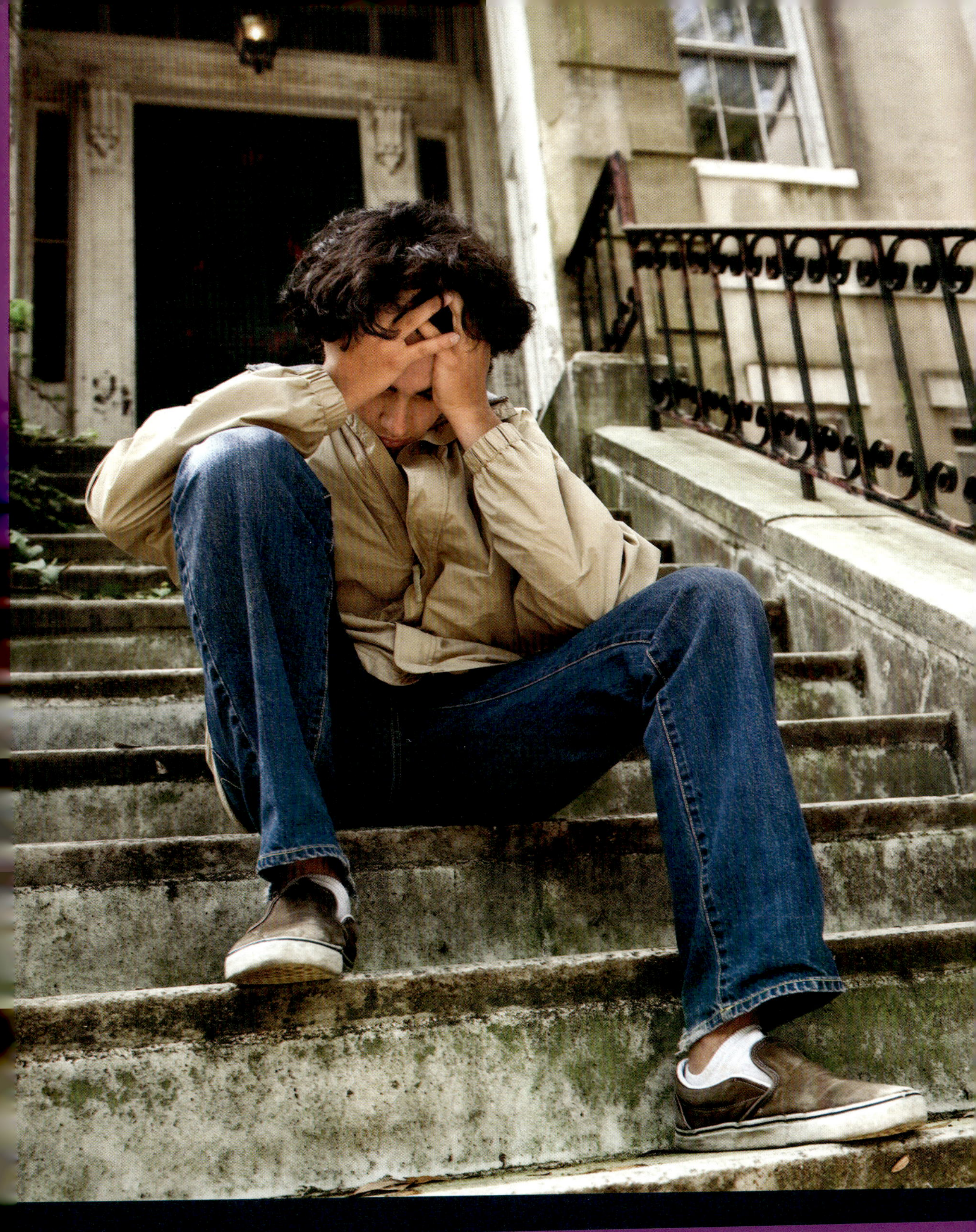

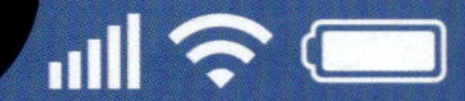

THE TRUTH ABOUT DRUGS

Drug addiction can happen for different reasons. Some people get addicted to pills given to them by their doctors for pain or **anxiety**. Others are addicted to illegal drugs they take for pleasure.

There are 7.4 million Americans who are addicted to illegal drugs.

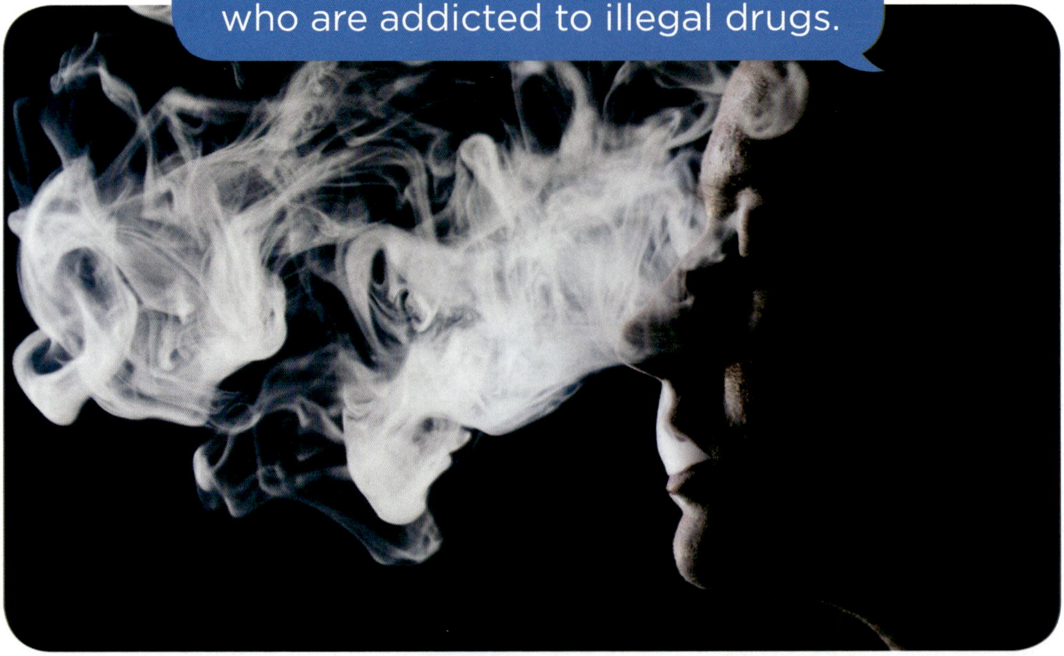

WHAT DO DRUGS DO?
Drugs change the way the body works.

ARE ALL DRUGS DANGEROUS?
Any drug can be dangerous. Certain drugs, like medicines, can be very helpful when needed if you follow a doctor's directions.

WHY ARE SOME DRUGS ILLEGAL?
Some drugs can hurt or kill the people who use them. They can also make people act strangely and cause harm.

CAN I TRUST THE DRUGS I TAKE?
Usually you can trust drugs you get from a **pharmacy** as long as you follow the instructions. You never know if you can trust drugs you get from other places.

Opioid, cocaine, methamphetamine, and **nicotine** addictions are some of the hardest to shake. They can also develop, or grow, very quickly. Drugs like marijuana are somewhat less addictive. But they can lead to addictive habits over time.

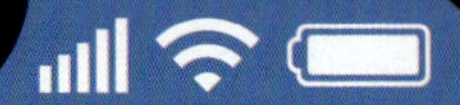

NICOTINE AND TOBACCO

There are 50 million Americans who are addicted to nicotine, a drug found in tobacco. Nicotine gives a mild pleasant feeling. People take in the drug through cigarettes, cigars, vaping devices, snuff, and chewing tobacco. Nicotine is very addictive. The chemicals in tobacco cause terrible health problems over time.

More than 8 million people die each year from diseases due to tobacco use.

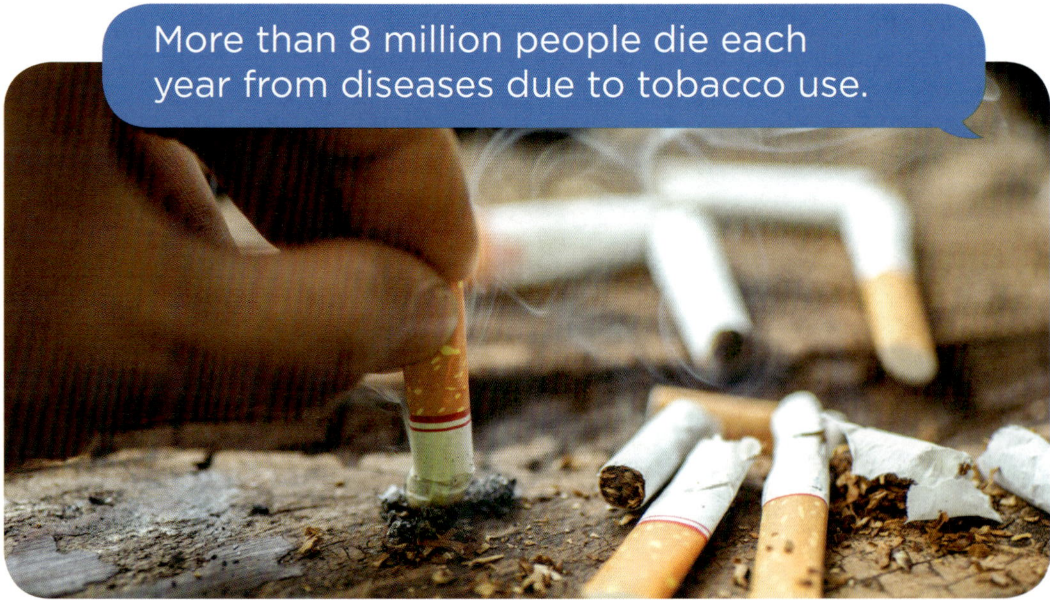

The younger a person is when they start using nicotine, the harder it is for them to stop. If you're having trouble with nicotine, it is important to seek treatment. Otherwise there is a very high risk of developing a disease.

Health Risks from Smoking Tobacco

- Cancer (30% of all cancer cases are connected to tobacco)
- Diabetes
- Lung diseases
- Vision issues
- Duller senses
- Teeth and gum disease
- Heart and blood pressure problems

Health Risks from Smokeless Tobacco

- Cancer of the mouth and throat
- Nicotine poisoning
- Heart disease
- Stroke

Health Risks from Vaping Nicotine

- Faster addiction
- Lung diseases
- Higher blood pressure
- Lung injuries

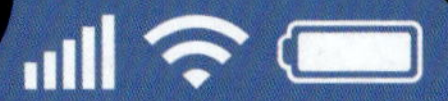

MARIJUANA

Marijuana, also known as pot or weed, is legal for adults in certain states. It also has some medical purposes. Using marijuana regularly can make it become an addictive habit. In some cases, illegal marijuana products used in vaping have made people die unexpectedly.

Some marijuana users have problems with memory, learning, and attention. The drug can be very dangerous for developing brains. In young people, marijuana is linked to **depression**, anxiety, and **schizophrenia**.

The chemical in marijuana that causes hallucinations is called THC.

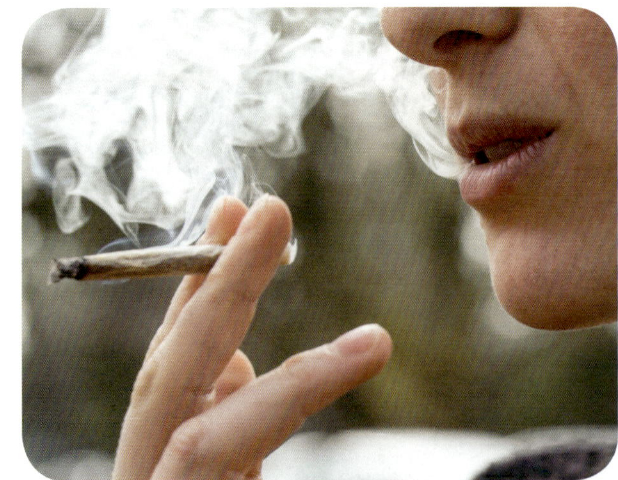

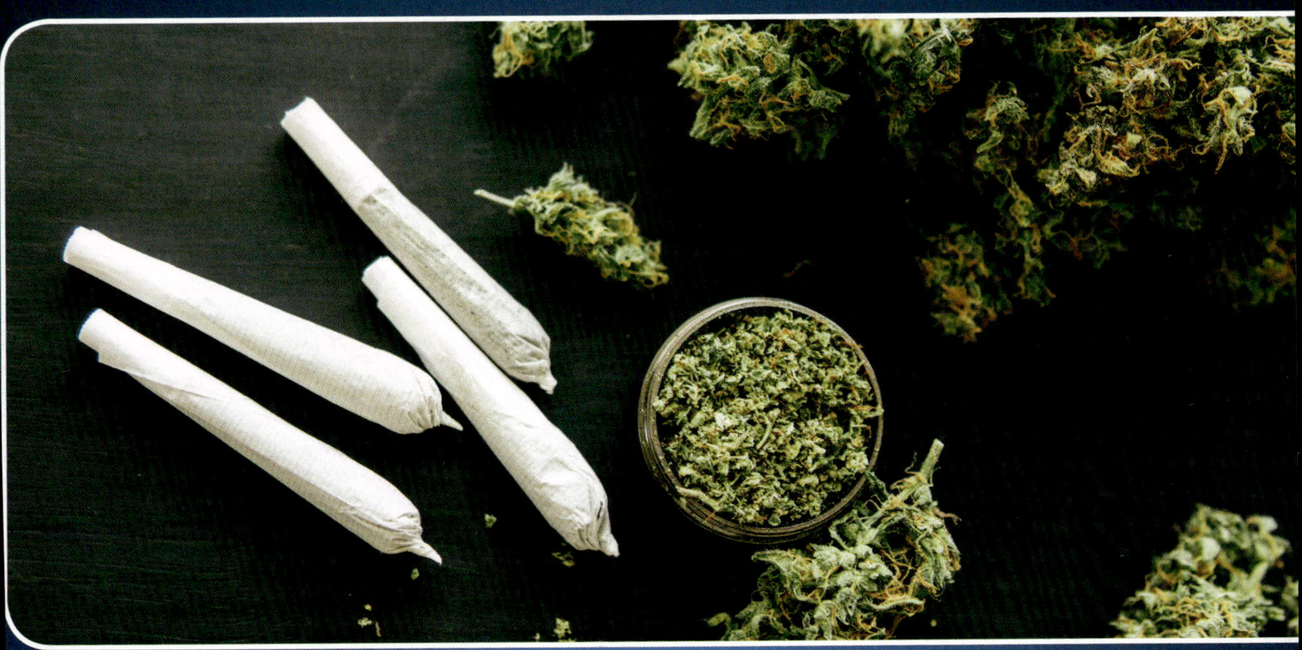

FACTS ABOUT MARIJUANA

- Of people who began using marijuana as teenagers, 1 in 6 are now addicted to the drug.
- Marijuana can lead to frightening experiences, especially at higher doses.
- While high on marijuana, the heart beats much faster.
- When smoked, marijuana can hurt the lungs like tobacco does.
- Marijuana is considered a **hallucinogen** and can change someone's sense of reality.
- Food products with marijuana in them are usually stronger and have longer-lasting effects than marijuana that is smoked or vaped.

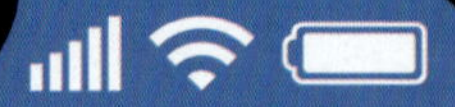

PAINKILLERS AND OPIOID ADDICTION

Some of the deadliest drugs in the world today are painkillers known as opioids. These are sometimes given to people by doctors after surgeries or injuries. They are extremely addictive.

Examples of opioids you might get from your doctor are oxycodone (Oxycontin, Percocet, and Percodan) and hydrocodone (Vicodin, Lorcet, and Lortab). Some people who are addicted to these drugs end up using heroin or fentanyl later. All of these drugs can lead to overdoses. During an overdose, a person may stop breathing and die.

Of American heroin users, 80 percent were first addicted to opioid painkillers. Every day, 115 Americans die from overdosing on opioids.

What do I do if my friend overdoses?

Someone who has overdosed from opioids may be cold, unresponsive, and breathing slowly or not at all.

Call 911 immediately.

Naloxone (Narcan) can stop the effects of an opioid overdose. Police cars, ambulances, and even schools might have this product. You can also get Narcan at pharmacies in some states without a **prescription**.

A person who has overdosed may need rescue breathing. Learn how to do rescue breathing at https://www.sharecare.com/health/first-aid-techniques/how-perform-rescue-breathing.

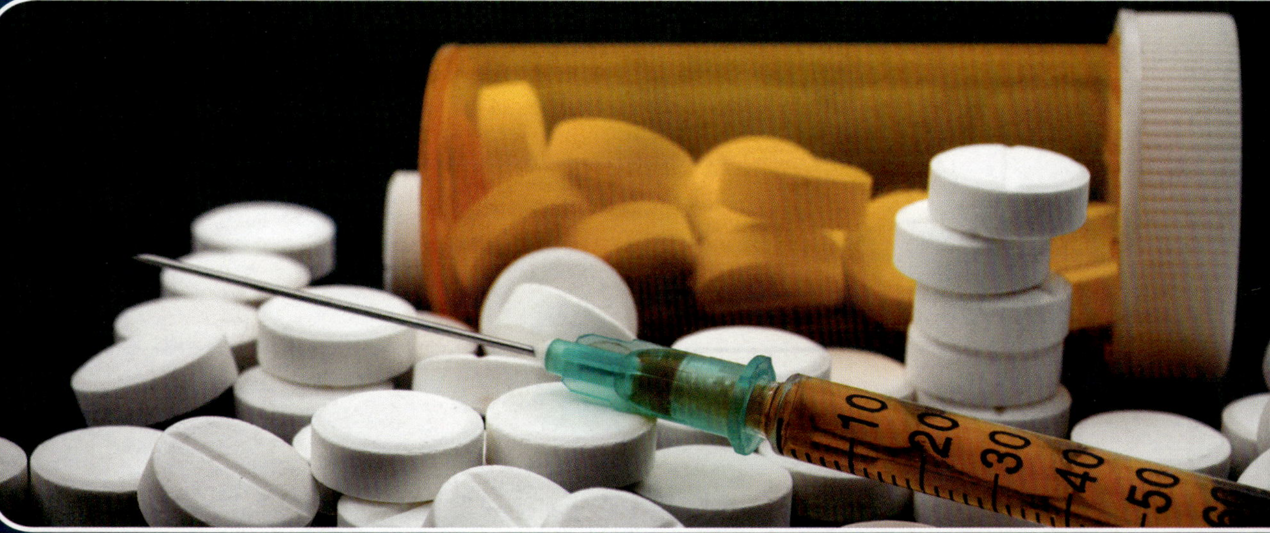

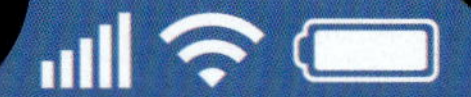

OTHER DRUGS

There are many different drugs you may come across. Unless you receive a drug from your doctor, you might not know for sure what it is. Even with medication, it is important to follow a doctor's directions. Otherwise you are risking addiction, disease, or even death.

Some street drugs are mixed with other, more dangerous, drugs. This has led to sudden deaths.

Like opioids, some **stimulants** and **tranquilizers** have medical uses. Many are also very addictive. Some can be deadly in high doses or when mixed with alcohol. While typically less addictive, hallucinogens sometimes cause scary experiences. They may make users hurt themselves or others. They can also harm developing brains.

You might have heard about some of the drugs below. None of them are safe without a doctor's prescription.

Hallucinogens/Psychedelics

DMT, DXM (robo), ibogaine, LSD (acid), magic mushrooms, MDMA (ecstasy/Molly), mescaline, ketamine (Special K), PCP (angel dust), salvia

Stimulants/"Uppers"

Adderall, anabolic steroids, cocaine/crack, MDMA (ecstasy/Molly), modafinil, methamphetamines (speed, ice, crystal meth), Ritalin

Tranquilizers/"Downers"

Ativan, Klonopin, Librium, Rohypnol, Valium, Xanax

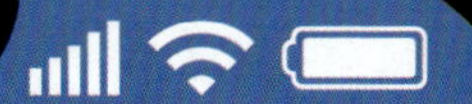

DRUG ADDICTION RESOURCES

If you, your friends, or family members have issues with drug addiction, don't be afraid to seek help. Contact these free resources:

National Drug Helpline

http://drughelpline.org
Call 1-844-289-0879 to speak to a caring counselor.

Partnership For Drug-Free Kids

https://drugfree.org/article/get-one-on-one-help
Text a message to 55753 for help regarding a family member struggling with drug addiction or call 1-855-378-4373.

Smart Recovery

http://www.smartrecovery.org/teens/
Find online meetings, messageboard discussion groups, and more.

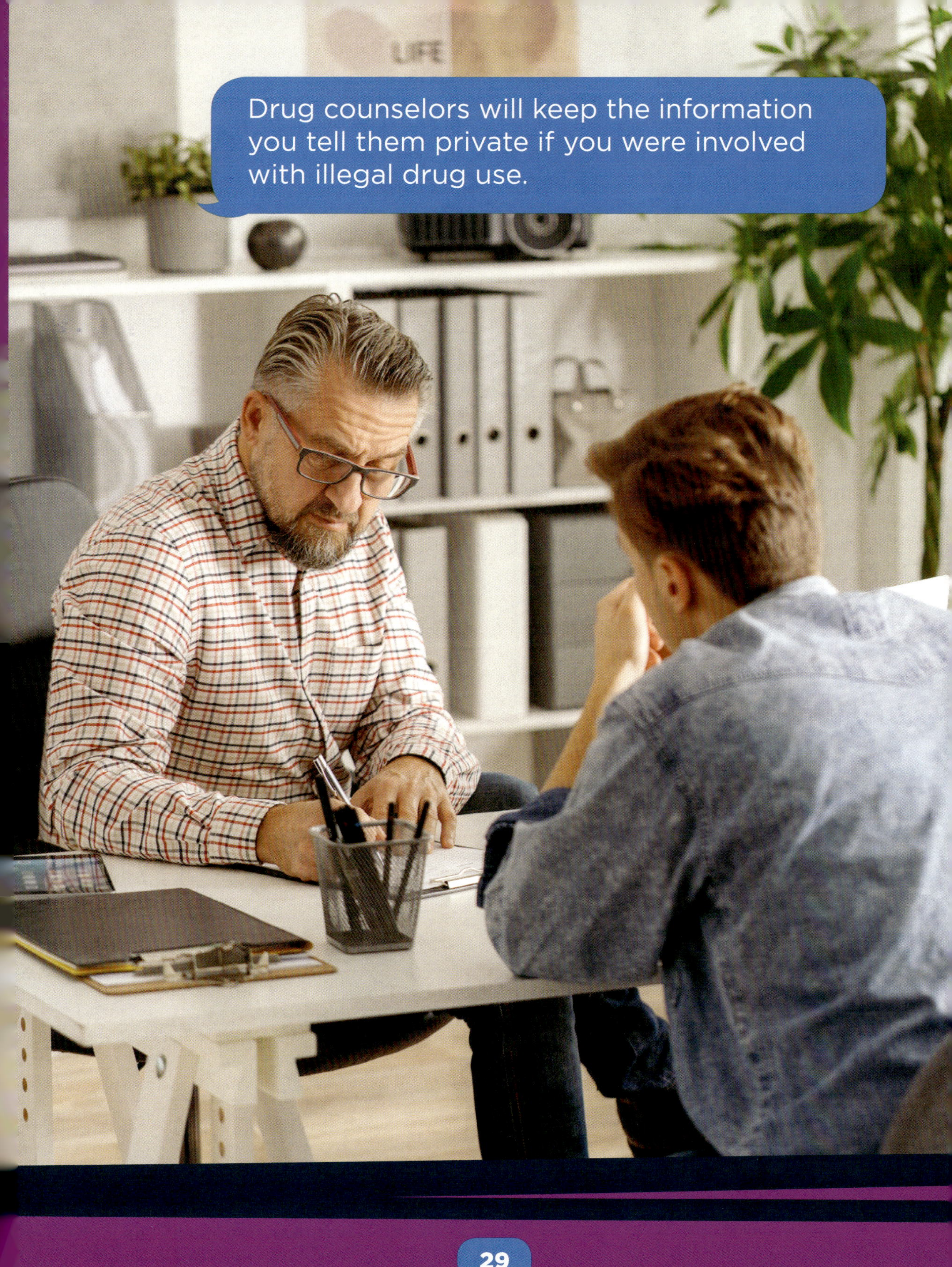

Drug counselors will keep the information you tell them private if you were involved with illegal drug use.

Chapter 4

TECHNOLOGY ADDICTION

I look at the clock. It's 3 a.m. Mom told me to go to bed hours ago. But I had to level my character up. Of course, I needed to buy new armor, too. I got caught up in a side quest during the game and then . . .

It's been the same story every night this week. I'm barely getting any sleep. I want to shut the screen off. But I feel so good right now. Why not forget about the morning? High school is pointless. I don't feel like I belong there. When I play video games, everything seems right. Life flows perfectly.

If only I wasn't tired all day. If only my grades weren't slipping . . .

About 10 percent of teens who play video games are addicted to gaming.

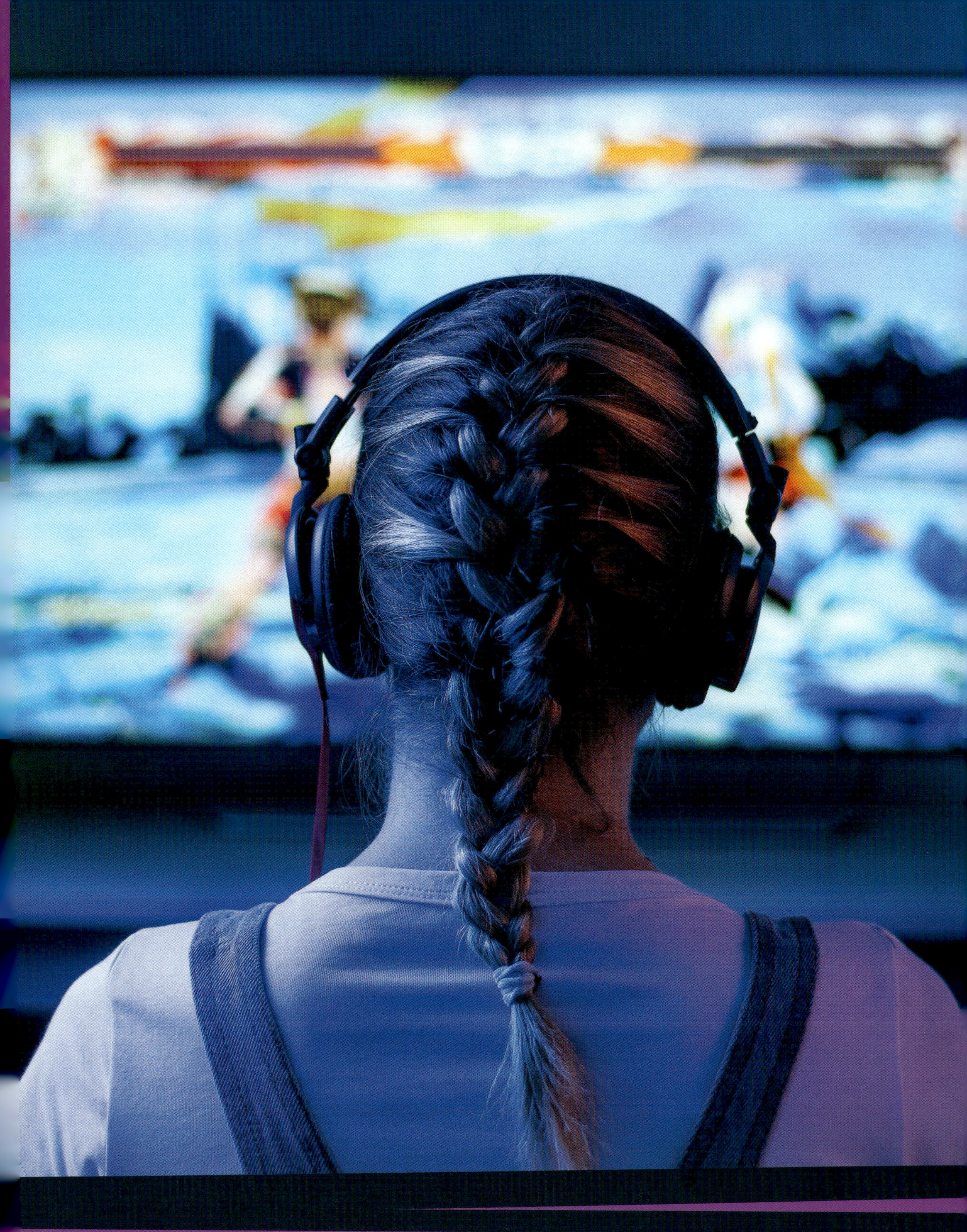

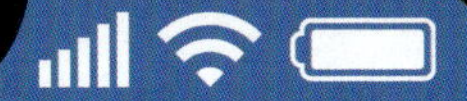

TAKING TECHNOLOGY TOO FAR

Each year brings with it new smartphones, televisions, and computers. In many ways, our devices make our lives easier. They keep us better connected. However, they can also create serious addiction problems.

People with Internet addiction disorder (IAD) show brain scans that look similar to individuals who have alcohol and drug addictions.

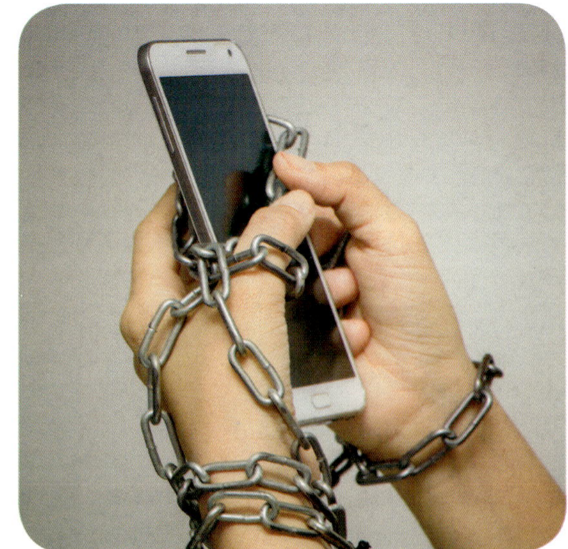

For teenagers, video games and social media can be especially addictive. Both provide ways of checking out of reality. They can help us cope with stress. They can also get in the way of daily life. They can keep us up at night. In the long run, this can make life even more stressful.

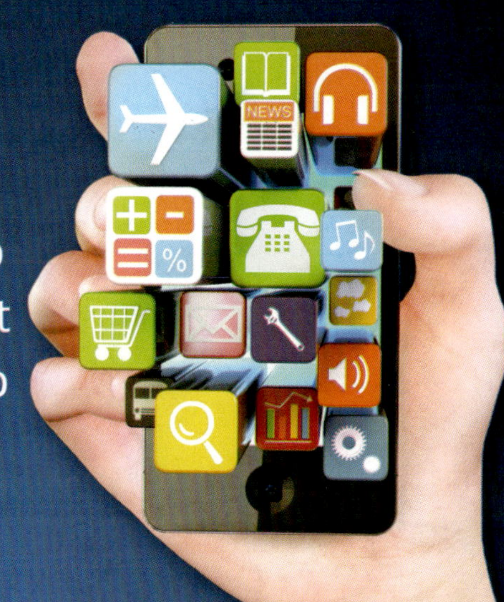

It's important to stay balanced when using technology. There are so many ways to get addicted.

Addiction can be caused by overusing:

- Apps and video games
- Gambling sites and fantasy sports
- Online pornography, or sex images and videos
- Social media, such as Instagram, Facebook, Reddit, Tumblr, Twitter, and Snapchat
- Text messaging
- YouTube, Twitch, and other online video channels
- Streaming services, like Amazon Prime, Disney+, Hulu, and Netflix

People addicted to technology can experience depression, anxiety, and powerful cravings when they are not using their devices.

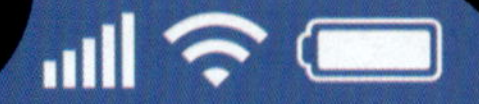

VIDEO GAME ADDICTION

Video game addiction is especially common among teenagers. Many people love playing games. But some take it to extremes. Those who are addicted to video games often don't get enough sleep. They cannot do the work they need to because of their gaming habits.

Role-playing games are considered the most addictive type of online game.

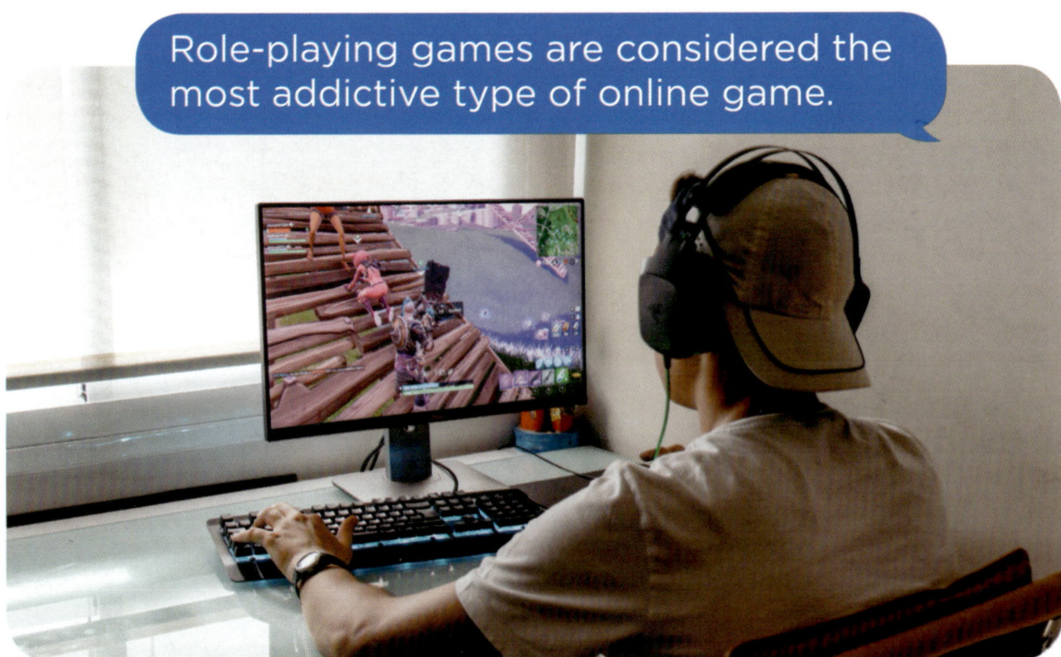

Online games are often the most addictive. Users are hoping to gain respect in a **digital** community. For some, this makes the digital world more important than life outside of gaming. More than 1 in 10 young gamers have trouble with video game addiction.

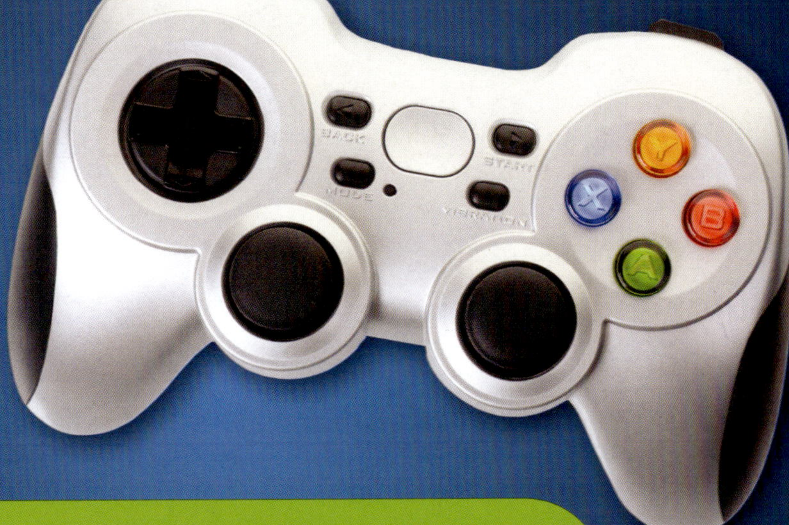

HERE ARE THE FACTS

- Some kids and teens have gone to rehab because they spend more than 12 hours each day playing games like *Fortnite*.
- People with video game addiction sometimes also abuse drugs and alcohol while playing.
- Video game addiction is connected to lower grades in school.
- The most helpful therapy for video game addiction is called cognitive behavioral therapy (CBT). It focuses on emotions and ideas people have.

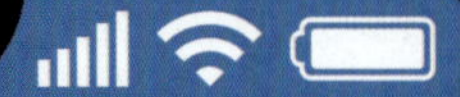

SOCIAL MEDIA ADDICTION

About 50 percent of teens say they spend too much time on their phones. One of the most addictive online areas is social media. People with social media addiction often have trouble sleeping. They may develop mental health issues.

Between 5 and 10 percent of Americans are addicted to social media.

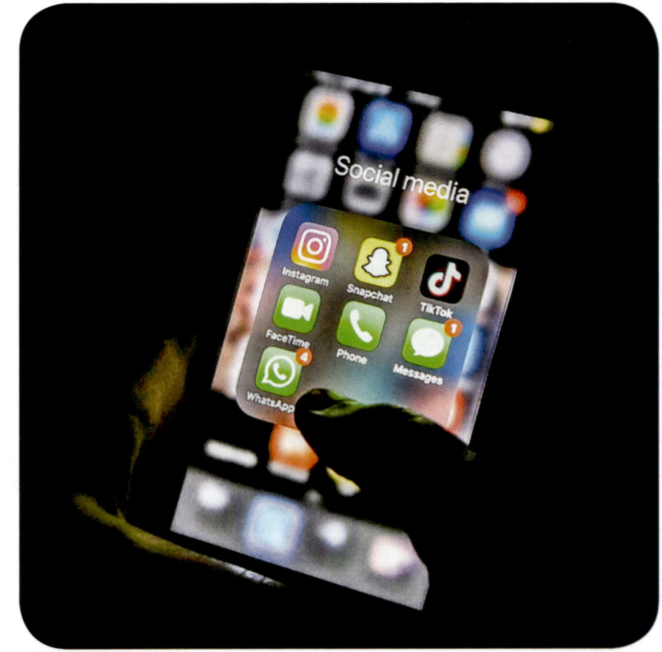

Social media and Internet communities can present risks and dangers. Teens sometimes engage in sexual behavior online. This can be dangerous or illegal. Certain Internet communities are violent or hateful. Bullying is a huge problem online. It can add to someone's depression, anxiety, or interest in suicide, or killing oneself.

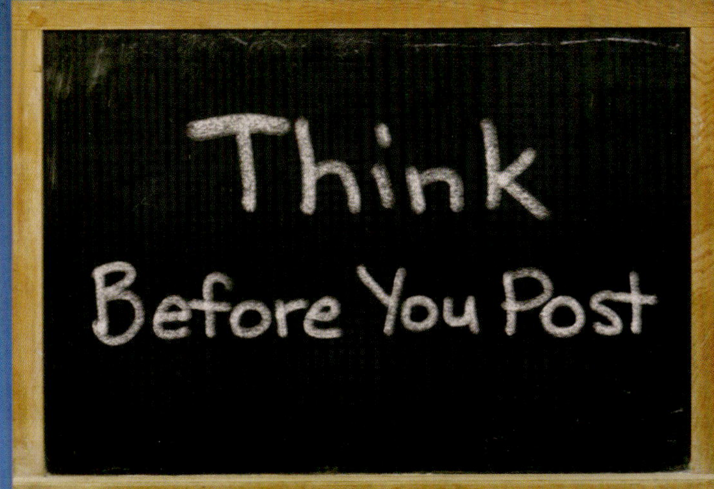

HERE ARE THE FACTS

- Likes, retweets, and happy emoticons create surges of dopamine in the brain. This can be very addictive.
- Teens who spend more than three hours a day on social media show higher levels of depression.
- People often experience low self-esteem because they compare themselves to others on social media.
- What people post on social media does not always show how they feel in real life.

TECHNOLOGY ADDICTION RESOURCES

Teens who are addicted to video games, social media, online pornography, or other technology-related issues can find help. Don't be afraid to reach out to people who care.

You don't need to feel trapped by the technologies you use!

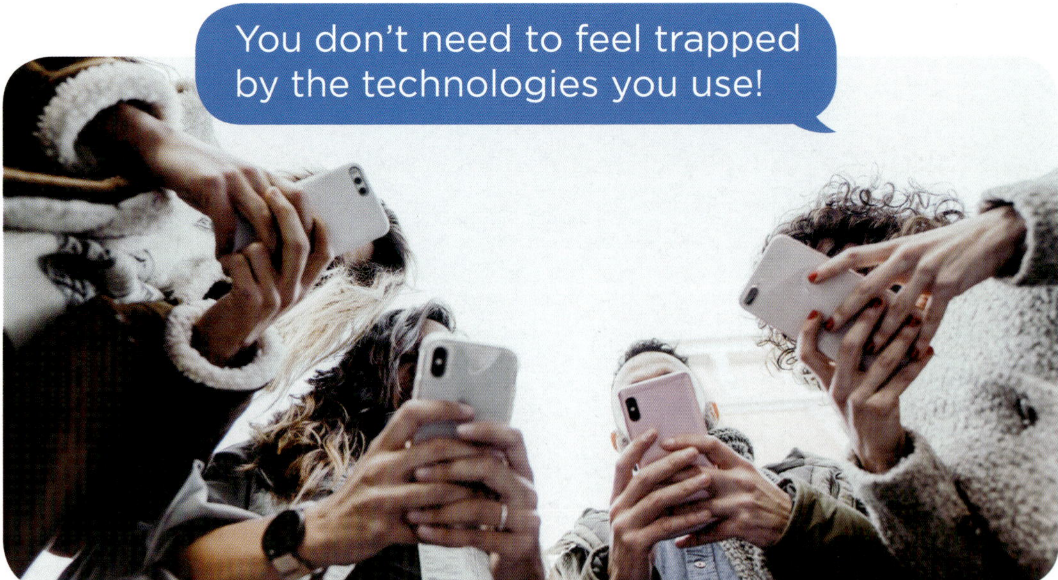

The Addiction Center

https://www.addictioncenter.com/

Contact 1-877-593-0639 to speak to an expert.

The Right Step Center

https://www.rightstep.com/rehab-blog/social-media-addiction-help

Call 1-844-768-0396 for help.

The Center for Internet and Technology Addiction

https://virtual-addiction.com/

Call 860-561-8727 for help.

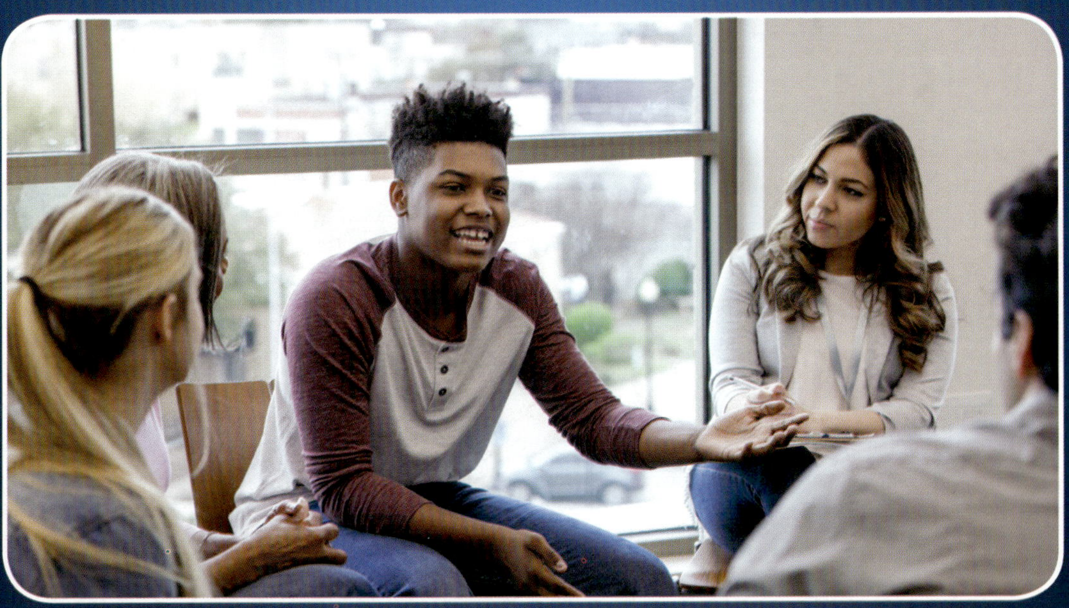

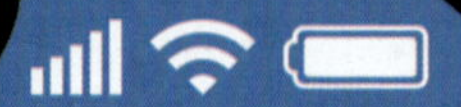

Chapter 5

OTHER TYPES OF ADDICTION

Addiction can sneak up in any area of life. It can even enter into parts of being human that no one can avoid. Some people, for example, struggle with food-related addictions. They might eat **compulsively** or have problems eating at all. This can affect their health and their self-esteem.

About 10 million Americans are considered gambling addicts. Some end up homeless or unemployed.

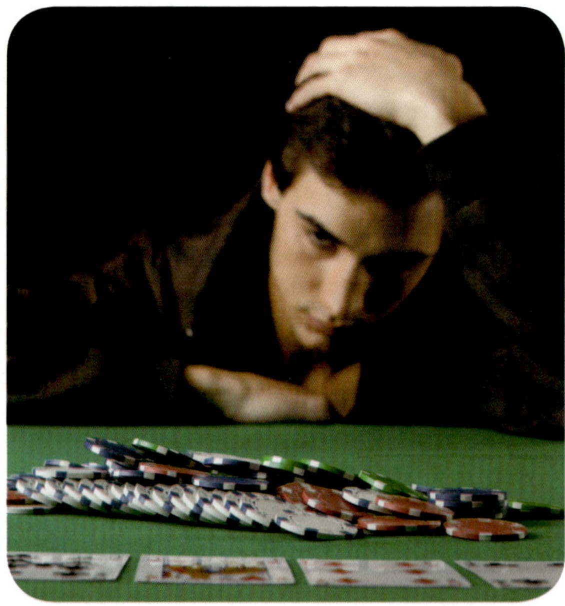

Another highly addictive activity is gambling. People who gamble too much sometimes fall into deep debt. They might spend all their money on their addiction. This could ruin their lives and tear their families apart.

OTHER COMMON SOURCES OF ADDICTION AND COMPULSION

- Cleaning
- Chewing ice
- Eating dirt
- Hoarding pets
- Pulling hair
- Shopping
- Tanning
- Thrills and risks
- Coffee
- Cutting and self-harm
- Exercise
- Plastic surgery
- Sexual behavior
- Stealing
- Tattoos and piercings
- Work

As you can see, addiction can show up anywhere—even in the things we love or have to do! While some of these addictions and compulsions might seem strange to outsiders, they are all more common than you might expect.

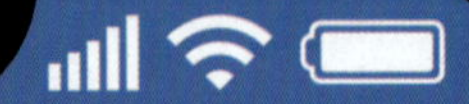

YOU ARE NOT ALONE

You don’t have to be ashamed if you, a friend, or someone in your family has a problem with addiction. It’s part of being human. We need to notice when our habits are hurting us and those we love. It’s important that we get help and support whenever we need it.

Many people who work as counselors or on crisis helplines have overcome addiction themselves. They might also have family members affected by addiction. They understand how painful or uncomfortable talking about the issue can be. You can trust them to help point you toward a brighter future.

ProjectKnow
American Addiction Centers

https://www.projectknow.com/how-to-help/teen/

Call 1-877-977-3727 for help.

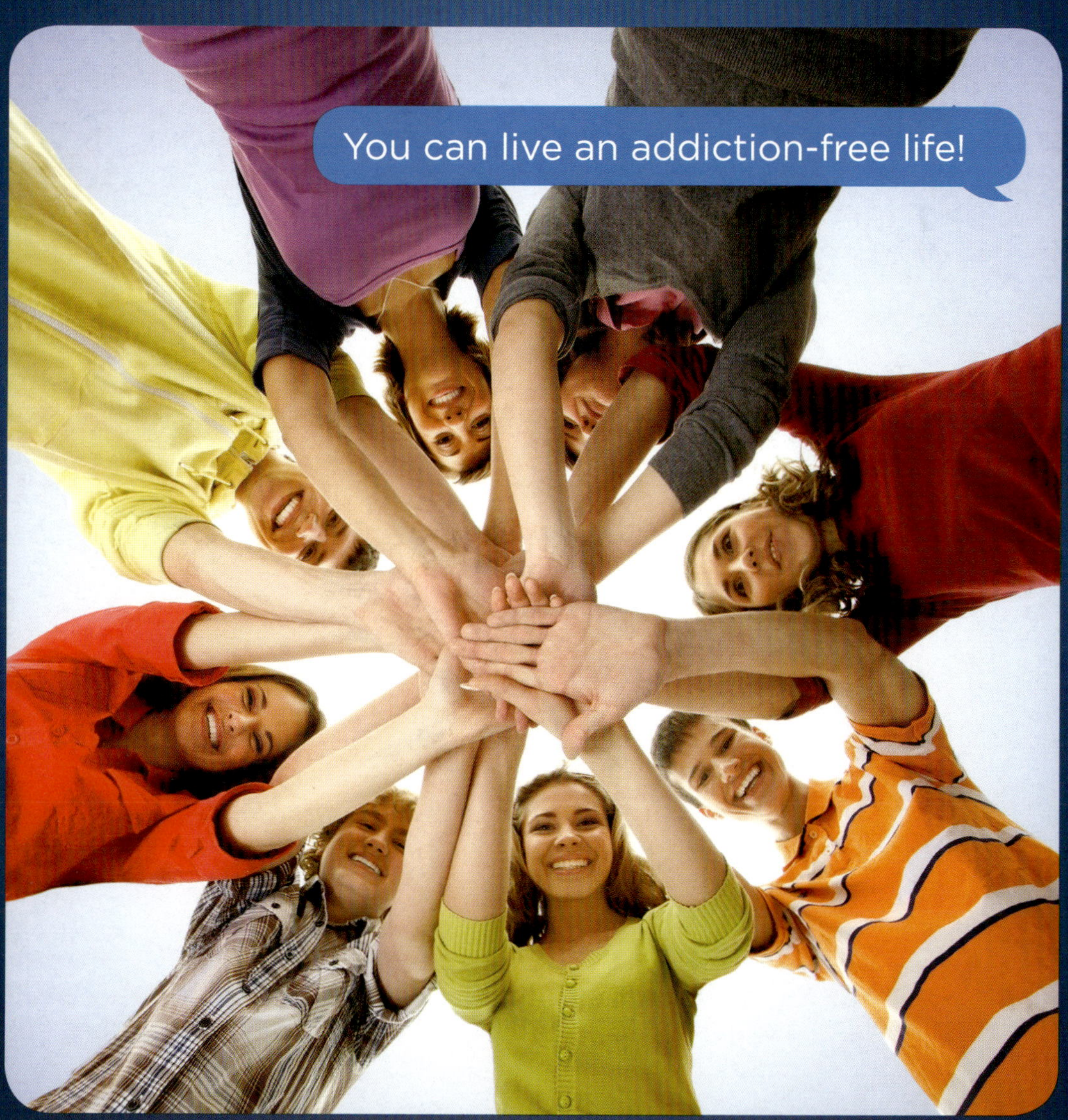

Chapter 6

A Fresh Start

I found out my friend Max will be getting the support he needs! He called a helpline and spoke with a counselor. Max will start treatment soon so he can live a healthier life. He already seems more connected to the world.

I'm grateful there are people out there who want to help. There are so many resources available for those who need them. I hope that Max can see just how much he matters to me. I am so happy he is taking a step in the right direction. There's so much life ahead for both of us!

More than 22 million Americans living today have recovered from addictions to drugs and alcohol.

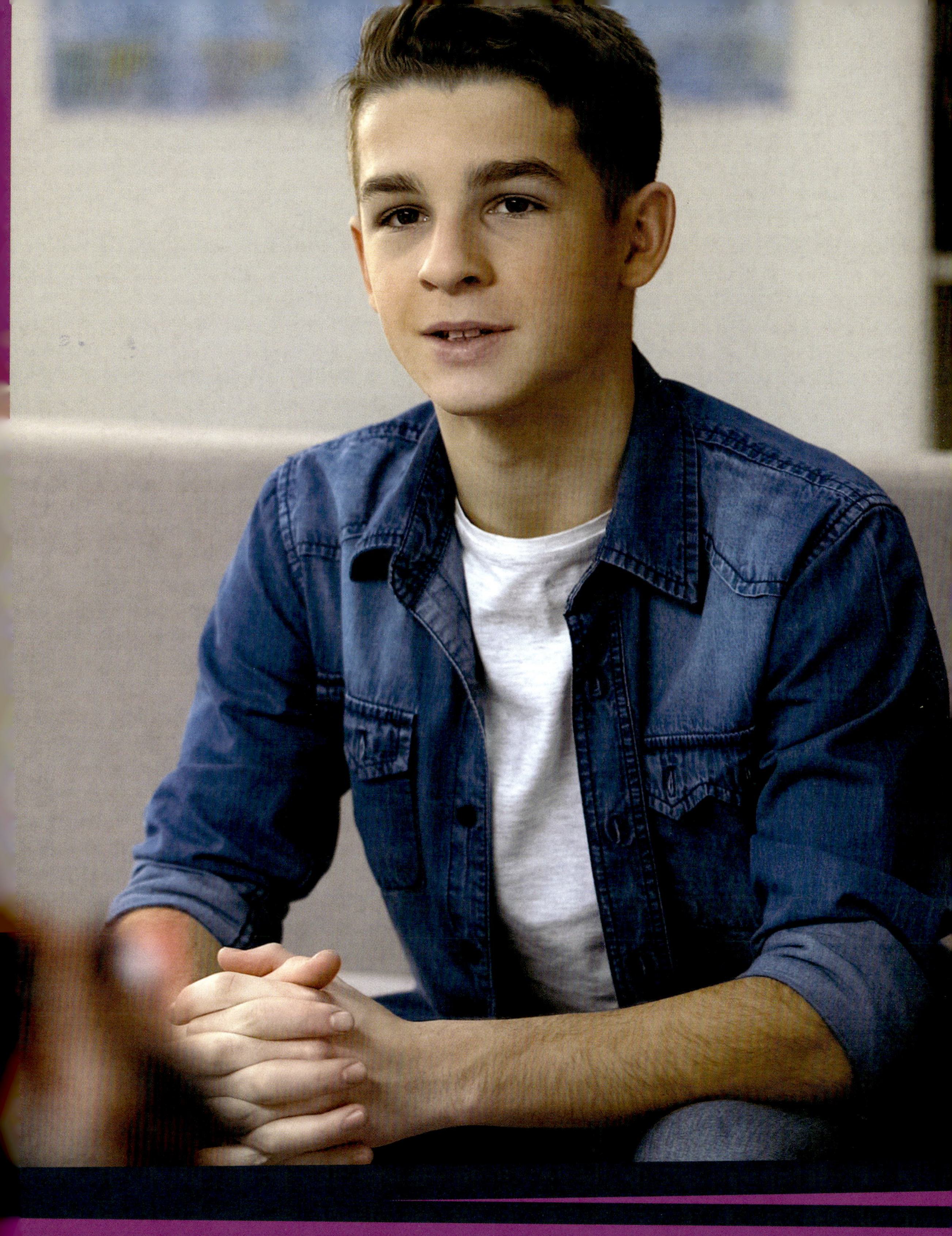

GLOSSARY

anxiety: A state or disorder involving fear or nervousness.

compulsive: Impossible to stop or control.

crisis: Emergency.

depression: A serious medical condition in which a person feels very sad, hopeless, and unimportant and often is unable to live in a normal way.

detox: A special treatment that helps a person to stop using drugs or alcohol.

digital: Related to computer technology.

dopamine: A chemical in the brain tied to pleasure, memory, learning, and movement.

hallucinogen: A drug that causes people to see or sense things that may not be real.

liquor: A strong alcoholic drink like vodka, rum, or whiskey.

nicotine: A poisonous substance in tobacco that makes it difficult for people to stop smoking cigarettes.

opioid: A type of drug used to treat intense or long-lasting pain.

pharmacy: A store or part of a store in which drugs and medicines are prepared and sold.

prescription: A written message from a doctor that officially tells someone to use a medicine or therapy.

rehabilitation: A program to bring a person back to a healthy condition after a drug or alcohol problem, injury, or illness.

reward circuit: A pathway in the brain related to pleasure and learned behavior.

schizophrenia: A very serious mental illness in which someone cannot think or behave normally and often experiences delusions.

sober: Not using drugs or alcohol.

stimulant: A drug that makes people more active or gives them more energy.

tranquilizer: A drug that causes people or animals to become very relaxed and calm.

trigger: Something that causes something else to happen.

INDEX